complexion perfection

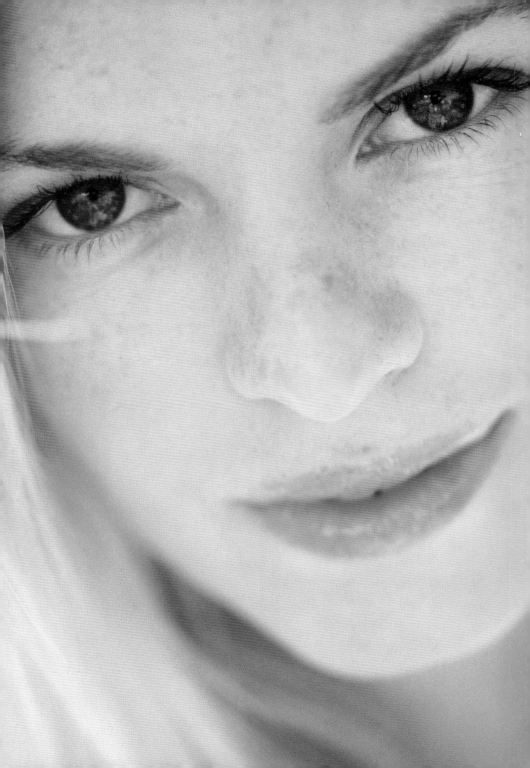

Wendy Lewis

complexion perfection

the lowdown on achieving spot-free skin

QUADRILLE

Editorial Director: **Jane O'Shea**

Creative Director: **Mary Evans**

Designer: **Sue Storey**

Project Editor: **Lisa Pendreigh**

Editor: **Katie Ginn**

Picture Research: **Nadine Bazar**

Illustrations: **Sue Storey**

Production: **Nancy Roberts**

First published in 2002 by Quadrille Publishing Limited
Alhambra House
27–31 Charing Cross Road
London WC2H OLS

Cataloguing-in-Publication Data: a catalogue record for this book is available from the British Library.

ISBN 1 903845 67 X

Printed and bound in Singapore

Contents

INTRODUCTION 6

THE BASICS 8

OIL PATROL 22

UNDERCOVER 36

AT THE CHEMIST 48

AT THE DOCTOR 58

SCAR WARS 76

BLUSHING BEAUTY 84

SUMMING IT UP 92

INDEX 94   ACKNOWLEDGMENTS 96

Great skin is the best accessory. It can make you look healthy and leave you bursting with vitality, and it makes you feel great about your appearance. Achieving smooth and clear skin is within everyone's reach. You just have to know what to do and what to avoid. Women crave information on the latest and greatest spot-reducing creams and acne remedies. Now, for the price of a lipstick, girls can get the real scoop on one of their top beauty concerns – pimples. This comprehensive guide delivers fresh solutions to the age-old problems of blemishes, oil-slicks, rosacea, cysts and blackheads, from the forehead down to the back – for prevention, maintenance and correction. It features the lowdown on the most state-of-the-art methods, what works and what's a waste of money, top clinical advances, new para-surgical treatments, DIY home remedies, as well as resources for how to find a good doctor, shopping guides and web links.

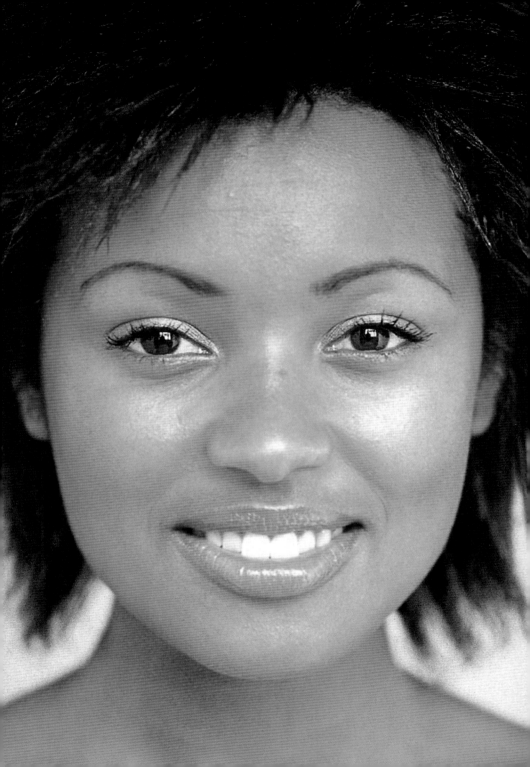

THE BASICS

THE BASICS

Hormonal and other internal upheavals have a way of leaving their mark on your skin, in the form of spots, skin eruptions and other lumps and bumps. Acne is the most common skin disease, but only 7 per cent of the 70 million sufferers ever see a dermatologist for help. Acne is a build-up of dried oil and dead skin cells in the hair follicles under the skin. Hormones, particularly male hormones called androgens, stimulate the hormone-sensitive sebaceous glands, which produce sebum. Like many other skin conditions, genetics play a part. All of these factors work together to start the vicious acne cycle.

If spots are a major problem in your life, join the club. Getting the odd spot is to be expected - we all have oil glands and sometimes they get clogged. The good news is that help is at hand. Whether you have the occasional flare-up or chronic acne that makes you want to hide, there are many effective treatment options. There's still no cure, with or without a prescription. The secret to controlling it is PREVENTION. Most acne therapies require ongoing treatment to keep your skin clear. Even after blemishes disappear, using an effective acne treatment will keep new ones from forming. The first step is determining the type and cause of your acne.

demystifying spots

Although spots come in a variety of forms, all pimples start out the same – as a plugged-up follicle. Acne actually begins 2–3 weeks before the blemishes show up on your face.

Blackheads

'open comedos' formed when dead skin cells and sebum are tightly packed inside a follicle where the walls have broken. If the plug enlarges and pops out of the duct, it's a blackhead. The skin cells and oil give it a dirty appearance that won't wash away, although it is not dirt. The colour is due to a build-up of melanin, the dark pigment in the skin.

Whiteheads

'closed comedos' where the plug stays below the surface of the skin so the follicle wall does not break. Whiteheads are formed on or under the skin and show up as a skin-coloured or slightly inflamed bump in the skin. A whitehead differs from a blackhead in that the opening of the plugged sebaceous follicle is closed or very narrow, instead of distended and open. With inflammatory acne, whiteheads become infected with bacteria, which causes them to swell.

Papules

red, raised bumps or inflamed lesions that occur when the oily materials inside the follicle rupture into the surrounding skin. They show up as small solid lesions of less than 5 cm in size, slightly elevated above the surface of the skin.

Pustules

dome-shaped, fragile lesions similar to papules but slightly more inflamed with visible pus that typically consists of a mixture of white blood cells, dead skin cells and bacteria. A pustule that forms over a sebaceous follicle usually has a hair in the centre. Pustules that heal without turning into a cystic form don't usually leave scars.

Cysts

a severe form of inflammatory acne, cysts are closed hard sacs that can be as large as marbles and very painful. A cyst is larger than a pustule and extends into the deeper layers of the skin where they can destroy tissue structures and cause scarring. Localized cystic acne is seen as a few cysts on the face, chest and back. Diffuse cystic acne affects wide areas of the face, chest and back. Systemic therapy with Isotretinoin is generally the only effective treatment.

causes

Hormones
Oil production
Follicle changes
Bacteria

Like many beauty afflictions, acne is
often linked with genetics and stress.
Adding hormones to the mix can really ruin your skin. Getting
to the root of the problem takes know-how and perseverance.

Hormones

Acne usually begins when the body starts to produce hormones called androgens. Hormones trigger most attacks, specifically androgens that are produced by the ovaries and adrenal glands in women. When androgen production goes into high gear between the ages of 11 and 14, acne can start to show up. Androgens cause the sebaceous glands to get larger. When they get over-stimulated, acne flares up. That's why you don't usually see acne before puberty. Although the peak years for females are ages 14 to 17, acne can show up any time your hormones are in flux, for example during pregnancy or the menopause. The odd pimple that shows up once in a while during your period is not necessarily acne.

Oil production

As the sebaceous gland is stimulated by androgens, it produces more oily sebum that accumulates in the follicle, and travels up the hair shaft to the surface of the skin. As it travels, it also mixes with normal skin bacteria and dead skin cells that have been shed from the lining of the follicle. The greater the oil production, the greater the likelihood that the hair follicle will become clogged and result in spots.

Follicle changes

As androgen production increases and sebaceous glands enlarge, the inner lining of skin in the hair follicle also changes. Normally, dead cells inside the follicle are shed, and get expelled onto the surface. During hormonal flux, these cells are shed more rapidly and tend to stick together. When they mix with sebum, they can clog the follicle and form a plug.

Bacteria

The clogged follicle becomes a breeding ground for bacteria. One type of bacteria is Progionibacterium acnes (*P.acnes*). *P. acnes* is on the skin even when there is no acne. When the sebaceous gland gets clogged and sebum builds up inside the follicle, *P.acnes* multiplies rapidly. Chemicals produced by the bacteria can cause inflammation in the follicle and surrounding skin.

Acne by prescription

Medications that may cause or aggravate acne include Testosterone, a male hormone and Gonadotrophin, used for pituitary disorders, anabolic steroids, taken by athletes to bulk up muscle and corticosteroids, which taken orally or applied topically to the skin can contribute to plugging up follicles. Acne may also be affected by anti-epileptic drugs, Lithium – a medication for bi-polar disorder, as well as Cyclosporin, used for post-transplant patients.

grading acne

Dermatologists grade acne in order to select the most appropriate treatment for you and to follow your progress along the way.

Not all acne is the same. It goes through stages and changes during the month, the season and the year. Everything is relative – what is considered 'a few' to some, may seem like 'a lot' to someone else. Even one persistent spot can seem like a lot if it's on your face.

Determining the severity of your acne is based on clinical observation. Acne does not begin at the appearance of a spot. That is the end result of the process. To decide what methods are best for your particular acne, dermatologists count the number of lesions of each kind on both sides of the face. If you can count more than 10 blemishes on your face consistently, your acne could be considered serious enough to seek out medical attention. Fortunately, the most common form is the mildest, and the least common is the most severe. Grade 2 is the most difficult to clear up. Size counts too – large inflamed pustules are more serious than tiny ones. When you get to Grade 4, doctors tend to bring out the heavy artillery – usually topical and oral medications – to get the job done, because nothing else will be effective.

BEAUTY BYTES:
To find an acne guru who can treat you, visit www.aad.org and www.bad.org.uk.

Making the Grade

Grade 1	Mild	A few scattered blackheads and whiteheads on each side of the face.
Grade 2	Mild to moderate	30–40 whiteheads that mature into blackheads
Grade 3	Moderate to severe	Considered 'active' acne, a mixture of whiteheads and blackheads on the face, some inflamed, and a few cysts.
Grade 4	Severe	3 quarters of the face is involved, chronic painful nodular cysts in addition to symptoms of Grades 1, 2 and 3.

Get to know the skin you're in. Keep a journal of your spot history. Check your face twice a month – before and after your period – and count the number of lesions, where they are, how large they are and if they are inflamed and red.

raging hormones

Once you've survived the awkward teenage years – braces, cramming for tests, bad school photos – you would expect to have left pimples and problem skin behind.

Not always. If you've been dealing with breakouts since your teens, you've probably heard things like 'Don't worry, lots of kids your age go through this.' or 'You'll grow out of it.' While millions of teenagers suffer before emerging clear skinned, others are not so fortunate. Sometimes it doesn't clear up after you leave school. It may not even start until adulthood. Perhaps you sailed through your teens with the perfect skin, only to start breaking out in your 20s, 30s or 40s.

REALITY CHECK:
Oily skin tends to develop lines and wrinkles at a slower rate and later age, so your oily skin may actually be keeping your skin looking younger for longer when it counts.

A staggering 4 million adults suffer from acne. Many cases begin in adulthood, often accompanying the hormonal changes of pregnancy, irregularities in the menstrual cycle or ovarian cysts, which may increase androgen productivity. Women typically suffer from adult onset or worsening acne more often than men, and they may have the problem for many years. Stress almost always plays a role because it stimulates the gland that produces androgens. When you feel stressed, your hormone levels fluctuate, which can cause increased oil production in the skin. Most of us notice an extra blemish or two before a major event in our lives.

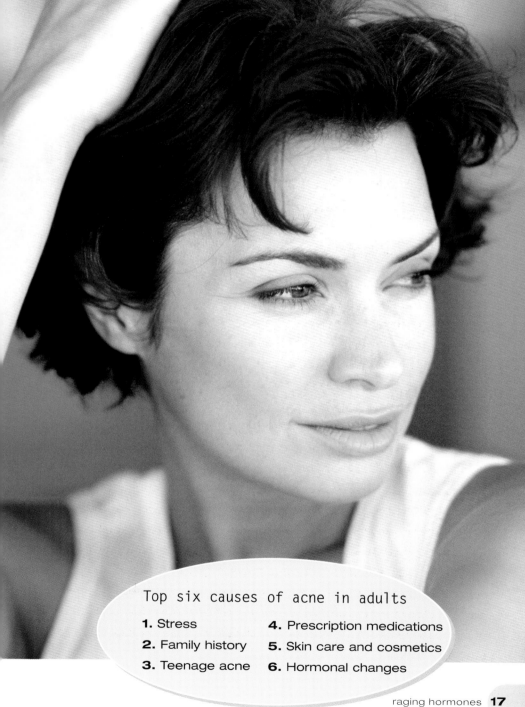

Top six causes of acne in adults

1. Stress
2. Family history
3. Teenage acne

4. Prescription medications
5. Skin care and cosmetics
6. Hormonal changes

spot cycle

Many women experience monthly acne outbreaks caused by the release of progesterone after ovulation.

Hormonal medications and endocrine disorders are also cited as causes of acne flare-ups in grown women. Even slight hormonal fluctuations can increase the number of new pimples, blackheads and whiteheads, as well as the oiliness of the forehead and cheeks. This is most common at about 5 days prior to the beginning of the cycle and remains for 7–10 days, so you should adjust your skin care regime to account for these monthly fluctuations.

The pill

Some women are genetically prone to drastic hormone swings, higher levels of androgens and oil glands that are more sensitive to hormones. Your doctor may recommend taking an oral contraceptive to change the balance between androgenic and female hormones and help control acne breakouts. Oral contraceptives that change a woman's hormone level can cause breakouts both when started and stopped. Some of the newer birth control pills are especially formulated to control acne, and one in particular, Ortho Tri-Cyclen®, has been approved by the US Food and Drug Administration for treatment of acne. This pill treats acne with a combination of ethinyl oestradiol, a synthetic oestrogen, and norgestimate, a progestin. Although the only specific oral contraceptive that has been studied clinically with regard to acne is Ortho Tri-Cyclen®, many dermatologists believe that any formulation with a low amount of androgen can be used to treat acne. The pill may not be effective at all, or only for a certain period of time. Improvement doesn't necessarily mean an end to complexion worries, but to some women, if their acne is better than it was, they're happy. The pill can be combined with other standard acne treatments like retinoids and antibiotics for maximum effectiveness. If your acne gets worse, other therapies will be needed. When bacteria enter into the picture and inflammation and redness become evident, more aggressive, whole body treatments such as oral antibiotics may be necessary. The pill can also have side effects including weight gain, blood clots, heart attack, stroke, hypertension and diabetes. These risks are higher in women who smoke and increase with age.

Your gynaecologist might suggest blood tests or an ultrasound to pinpoint any underlying hormonal imbalances that could be a contributing cause to your acne. Irregular periods, excess facial hair, oily skin and acne may be a sign of Polycystic Ovary Disease in which excess production of androgenic hormones may cause these effects.

BEAUTY BYTES:

For information about oral contraceptives and acne,

go to www.orthotricyclen.com

teen troubles

When your skin is spotty and shiny, you just feel like you want to hide. The best bet for teenagers is to take the fast track to oil control.

- Got blackheads? Get a Vitamin A derivative formula to get deep into oil plugs.

- Don't over coat your face with acne medications – use only a thin layer.

- If you can feel hard lumps deep under the skin, see a dermatologist. Don't self-treat.

- Less is more – don't overdo the scrubbing, massaging or cleansing.

- Try not to touch your face more than you have to. Hands can spread bacteria.

- Don't get discouraged if your treatment isn't working. Seek advice about switching.

- Once you find that magic combination that keeps your acne under control, stick with it.

- Work to keep skin balanced – a good ratio of oily to dry. Don't dry your skin out and don't over-moisturize.

pregnant pores

If you have a history of acne your skin may either improve or worsen when you are expecting a child. Acne can appear at any stage during pregnancy and may or may not clear up on its own after childbirth.

When you are pregnant, anything goes. Breakouts can show up on the face, chest, back or elsewhere. Random flare-ups can happen at any time, especially in the first trimester and may level off during the second. Although prenatal acne cannot be prevented, there are steps you can take to minimize breakouts. Keep your skin in good shape before and after becoming pregnant and practise early intervention. Keep it simple – during pregnancy skin reactivity changes a lot and your skin may be sensitive to certain ingredients. Some glycolic acid products are considered safe for use by pregnant women, but most common acne treatments are a no go. Whatever is done to the mother may affect the foetus. Medications like antibiotics, vitamin A derivatives and benzoyl peroxide, should not be used by pregnant women or resumed until the baby is weaned. Salicylic acid is not generally recommended, as it is absorbed through the skin and can interfere with blood clotting. These drugs fall under the US Food and Drug Administration 'Pregnancy Category C', meaning that animal studies have not been conducted and it is unknown whether they can harm the foetus or if the drug is excreted in human milk. The final decision should always be left to your obstetrician or paediatrician.

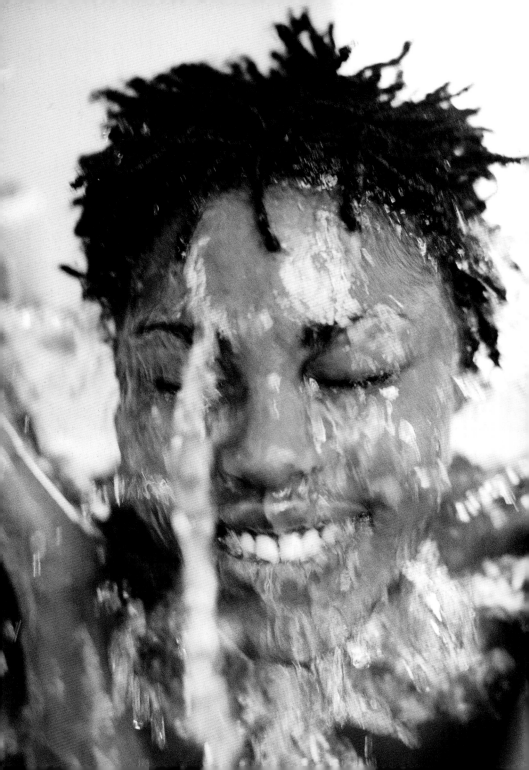

OIL PATROL

Forget what you've been hearing for aeons. The secret to reducing your shine lies more in what you put on your skin than what you put into your body. Contrary to popular myth, controlling oil glands is not food-related so following a strictly no-grease diet won't clear your skin. Gorging on chips, chocolate and other greasy foods may not cause acne, but won't do wonders for the way your clothes fit. Drinking lots of water won't really help acne either, even though it is good for you in other ways.

As with all things skin-related, go by what works for you. A few foods could present a problem. Some women swear they break out after consuming chocolate, ketchup, or cola. Avoiding allergenic substances such as dairy, caffeine and alcohol is sometimes recommended. Excessive iodine, found in fast foods, milk and shellfish has been cited as an acne trigger. If there might be a connection, it would be prudent to avoid foods that seem to aggravate spots, as a precaution. No one knows your skin like you do.

The same applies to skin care products, when you hit upon the right formula then stick to it. The trick is to eliminate excess shine without stripping the skin of its natural oils. Avoid any harsh products, instead choose cleansers, moisturisers and cosmetics specially formulated for oily skins. And remember, cleanliness is next to gorgeousness.

squeaky clean

You can't scrub spots away. Cleansing overload can actually aggravate pimples and slow down the healing process. The key to good cleansing is in using the correct products.

It is important to empty the pores of oil and fight the bacteria that cause the micro-infection which then turns into acne. It is natural to want to over-cleanse and over-exfoliate to wage war on every last drop of oil in the skin. This can trigger breakouts as oil glands will overcompensate. Acne doesn't necessarily mean your face is dirty. If you aren't washing thoroughly enough, dirt can clog pores and cause spots. But if you are constantly stripping away essential oils that your skin can't replace, you may be drying out the surface layer and making your skin less able to hold its own moisture. If your skin is dry, it will produce more oil, which is more likely to become trapped in your pores. Don't use soap – it can dry out the skin. Washing gently with a small amount of soap-free, scent-free cleanser is best. Abrasive cleansers and harsh exfoliants can aggravate acne. Wash your face from under the jaw to the hairline. Thoroughly rinse to get rid of any film from the cleanser. Astringents should only be used on oily areas, or if your skin gets shiny or doesn't feel clean without them.

TOP TIP:
Always use a fresh washcloth to avoid bacteria that can grow in damp cloths.

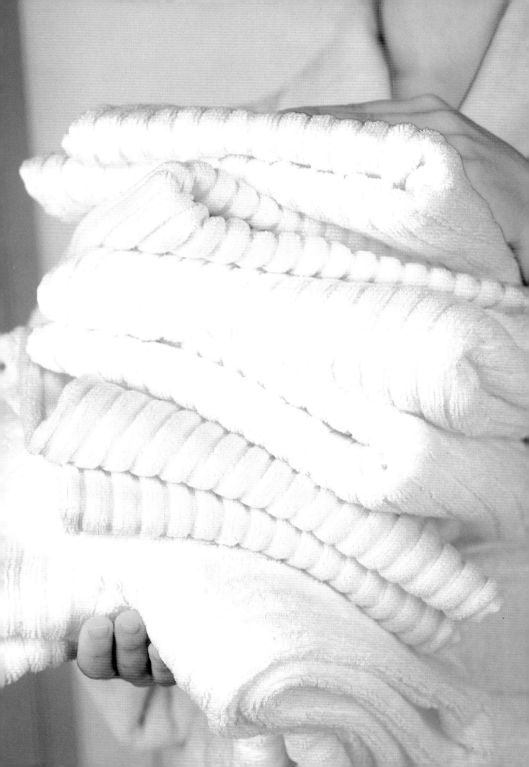

balancing act

Acne and dry skin can co-exist on the same face. Acne treatments tend to be very drying, especially if you have dry skin or eczema to start with. The key is to strike a balance.

Dry skin indicates that it is lacking oil, whereas dehydrated skin means a lack of water. Oily skin can be dehydrated even though it has plenty of oil. If you attempt to strip skin of all its oil content, you may end up with skin that is even oilier. Try a gentle, non-creamy cleanser and an oil free moisturizing product. Look for words like 'mild', 'non-irritating' and 'non-drying'. Be careful with cleansers that contain medications like salicylic acid. For best results, cleanse first, then apply your medication so you don't layer up, as this can add to irritation.

Terrible T-Zone

The T-Zone is the area of the face that runs from the forehead, down the nose, to the chin, where oil glands are most plentiful. Some surface grease on the skin is normal. It has the job of lubricating the skin's outer layer and keeping it protected. Most people who suffer from excess grease see the bulk of it on the forehead and nose. This just happens to be the most common location for acne. Your forehead oil will be reduced by most acne treatments. Humidity and high temperatures can wreak havoc on your T-zone as well, leaving it shiny. If you're active and enjoy sports, exercise and perspiration may cause excessive shine.

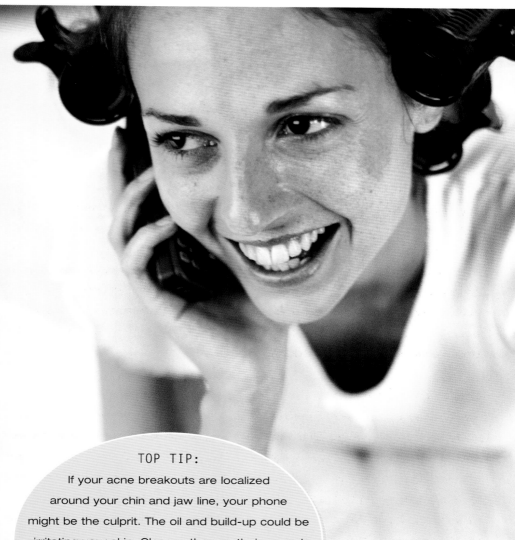

TOP TIP:

If your acne breakouts are localized around your chin and jaw line, your phone might be the culprit. The oil and build-up could be irritating your skin. Cleanse the mouthpiece and receiver every morning with hydrogen peroxide or alcohol. Don't let the phone rest between your chin and shoulder and keep it away from your skin.

tackling outbreaks

*Your first course of action is to treat breakouts on your own.
Review what you are currently using. Your skin care regime
may actually be the culprit.*

Choose products specially designed for oily skin types so they won't clog
pores. Whatever you do, declare a moratorium on any product that feels
creamy, heavy or isn't oil free. Women who are nearing 40 may feel inclined
to focus on moisturization and as a result, overload their skin with pore-
clogging potential. Gels or lighter lotions are better suited to oily skin. Blotting
out the oil, soaking it up and keeping shine-free can be a full-time job. Many
moisturizers, creams and other skin care and cosmetic products contain
fats, oils and waxes that can clog pores and make problem skin worse.

More women are seeking anti-acne treatments than ever before.
Current worldwide sales of both prescribed and over-the-counter acne
products are record-breaking. Anti-ageing creams used to be the prime skin
care products for adults. While the demand still increases steadily, women
now have an insatiable appetite for new and improved acne treatments.
Every acne sufferer has encountered over-the-counter products that only
work for a short while. The popular products work differently for each of us
because everyone's skin is different. The best-selling anti-acne systems
are designed to combat mild to moderate acne while also rejuvenating and
refreshing the skin. The most important products to include in your regime
are a mild cleanser, revitalizing toner, drying lotion and refining mask. By
improving the way dead skin cells exfoliate, they can't clog pores.

Exfoliation is king when it comes to skin care for oily, acne-prone skin types. First, figure out if your skin thickness is thin, medium or thick by judging its strength, resiliency, and general condition. Healthy skin is smooth, firm, tight, even, and has good tolerance levels. If your skin is fragile, you need to increase skin thickness by stimulating it to produce new collagen – which is what Retin-A® does. Thick skin needs to get sloughed to keep its barrier function intact. Look for more active concentrations (8 per cent or higher) of glycolic, lactic and beta hydroxy acid or salicylic acid, to produce a superficial glow and keep pores unclogged. If your skin can tolerate higher concentrations (10–15 per cent), they will work faster.

TOP TIP:
An oil-free product can become oil-based when it comes into contact with the natural oils in your skin and environmental debris.

Women with acne often need to change some of the cosmetics they use. All cosmetics should be oil-free. Lip products that contain moisturizers may cause small open and closed comedos to form. Hairstyling products that come into contact with the skin along the hairline can cause burning or stinging in people with acne. Hair dyes that contain coal tar have been cited as potential triggers. Other lesser known irritants include fabric softeners, cologne and hair spray. Choose formulas that are non-acnegenic – won't cause acne, pustules or papules, and non-comedogenic – won't cause comedos, blackheads or whiteheads. Some women find that even products labelled as non-comedogenic may cause acne.

the light stuff

Acne-causing ingredients show up in almost every skin care product in one form or another. It is difficult to find formulas that don't have any at all.

Everyone responds differently to each ingredient, so one woman could be using a cocoa butter based moisturizer and never break out, whereas for another woman, cocoa butter may prove disastrous. The concentration of each of these ingredients also has a bearing on how clogging they become. Some normally comedogenic ingredients may be fine in a low concentration. That's where the process of trial and error comes in.

The size of your pores is genetically determined. Nothing has been proven to permanently shrink them. Keeping pores clean and unplugged can make them look smaller. Pore strips may appear to be helping, but they really can't go deep enough to extract the gunk that's buried. You can prevent the keratinised plug from forming, with good exfoliation. Masks that contain kaolin, calamine or clay, will absorb excess oil, calm the skin and keep pores toned.

If enlarged, open pores are a real problem, the best way to tighten them is with a series of resurfacing treatments like superficial acid peels, micro-dermabrasions and non-ablative lasers. The added bonus is that these treatments are also great for fine lines and wrinkles.

The table opposite indicates how likely the listed ingredients are to clog pores, using the comedogenic scale. Those with a scale of 3 have the highest potential to cause problems.

Pore clogging ingredients

Ingredient	Comedogenic Scale	Ingredient	Comedogenic Scale
Lanolins		Acetlyated Lanolin	2
PEG 16 Lanolin	2	Ethoxylated Lanolin	3
Acids, Esters & Ethers		Isodecyl Oleate	2
Laureth 4	1	2-Elyhyl Hexyl Palmitate	2
Isopropyl Myristate	1	PPG2 Myristyl Propionate	2
Myristyl Myristate	1	Disodium Monocleanido PEG	2
Isopropyl Isotearate	1	Sulfosuccinate	2
Steareth 10	2		
Alcohols, Glycols, Sugars		Cetearyl Alcohol - Cetearth 20	2
Hexadecyl Alcohol	1	Sorbitan Sesquinoleate	3
Oleyl Alcohol	2	Glyceryl Stearate SE	3
Natural Oils		Soya bean Oil	3
Cocoa Butter	2	Wheat Germ Glyceride	3
Coconut Butter	2	Sulfated Castor Oil	3
Sesame Oil	3	Cotton Seed Oil	3
Avocado Oil	3	Sandalwood Seed Oil	3
Pigments		D&C Red #36	3
D&C Red #30	3		
Detergents		Sodium Lauryl Sulfate	2
Vitamins & Herbs		Tocopherol	3
PG Monostearate	3		
Waxes		Sulfated Jojoba Oil	3
Miscellaneous		Xylene	2

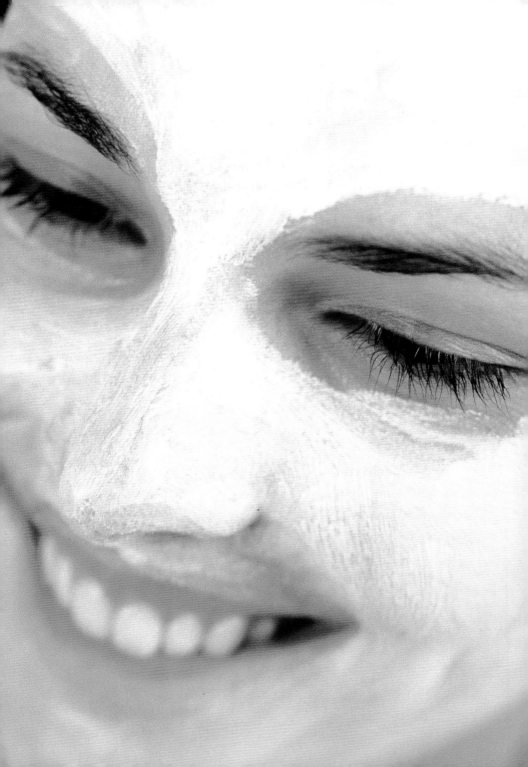

dos and don'ts for perfect skin

- **DO** keep your skin very clean with a series of facials from a beauty therapist to clean out pores.

- **DO** use a clay-based mask treatment once a week to eliminate excess oiliness.

- **DO** cleanse skin gently with a cleanser that doesn't leave a residue.

- **DO** avoid rough scrubbing and massage as this can stimulate glands.

- **DON'T** pick or squeeze pimples. This can spread infection and cause scarring.

- **DO** rinse with cold water after cleansing and use an alcohol-free toner or witch hazel.

- **DO** use a fresh washcloth daily to avoid bacteria that can grow in damp cloths.

- **DO** shampoo hair frequently, avoiding heavy cream rinses.

- **DON'T** let hair hang over your face, even at night, as this can spread oil.

- **DO** wash your face after exercising to remove sweat and dirt.

- **DON'T** keep touching your face as this will spread the bacteria that cause acne.

- **DO** use sunscreen containing an SPF15, Titanium Dioxide and Micronized Zinc.

big squeeze

Keeping your hands off your face serves two purposes: it prevents the spread of the bacteria that cause spots and it helps you resist the temptation to squeeze.

Squeezing forces infected material deeper into the skin, causing additional inflammation that takes longer to heal. Picking at spots will not help clear them up and may in fact leave you with permanent scars. Tissue injured by squeezing can become infected by staphylococci, streptococci and other skin bacteria. Popping zits can also injure the sebaceous follicle and the tissue around it, and force contents of the blackhead deeper as well as extruding it to the skin's surface. The result can be the start of an inflammatory reaction. Left on their own, blackheads do not usually get inflamed.

Squeezing or picking whiteheads is potentially even more harmful because they are more likely to become inflamed. Microcomedos are almost too small to be seen, but you can feel them as roughness on the skin. Once they become inflamed, they may develop into a pustule or a papule. Squeezing a microcomedo or closed comedo (whitehead) will not get the contents out anyway. A microcomedo is an undeveloped comedo, so there is really nothing there to squeeze out. A whitehead has such a small follicular opening that it is practically invisible, so little or no contents can be extruded. True cysts are nodules that rest deep below the skin's surface, so you can't get to them by squeezing yourself. Any attempt to manipulate them by squeezing or picking will just aggravate the inflammatory process.

saving face

There may not be much that can be done to stop the odd spot from appearing, but we can help to keep scars at bay by adhering to.a few simple rules.

Never squeeze your skin hard enough to leave an imprint. Don't apply concealer on blemishes that are open from squeezing or accidental scratching. They need to heal over before you can cover them up. If you have an open spot, apply an acne drying gel or lotion and then let it run its course. One of the causes of scarring and delayed healing is skin fragility. Using your fingernails to pick can strip away pigmented cells from the deep layer of the skin and leave you with a very uneven skin tone in desperate need of blending and bleaching. Be very careful about manipulating or picking away at areas of skin that are most prone to scarring – like the chin, chest and back.

Darker skin types are even more susceptible to scarring and 'post inflammatory hyperpigmentation' – doc-speak for dark blotches that often show up on Asian, Mediterranean and black skin types after acne lesions heal, and seem to take forever to clear, if at all. When melanocytes, which form the original colour of the skin, get disrupted, the skin needs outside help to come back to its normal state. This help usually comes in the form of exfoliating and bleaching agents like Tretinoin, Hydroquinone and Alpha and Beta hydroxy acids, to effectively lighten darkened areas so they blend in with the rest of your complexion. Total sun protection is a must for dark spots, as sun exposure will turn them darker and make them last longer.

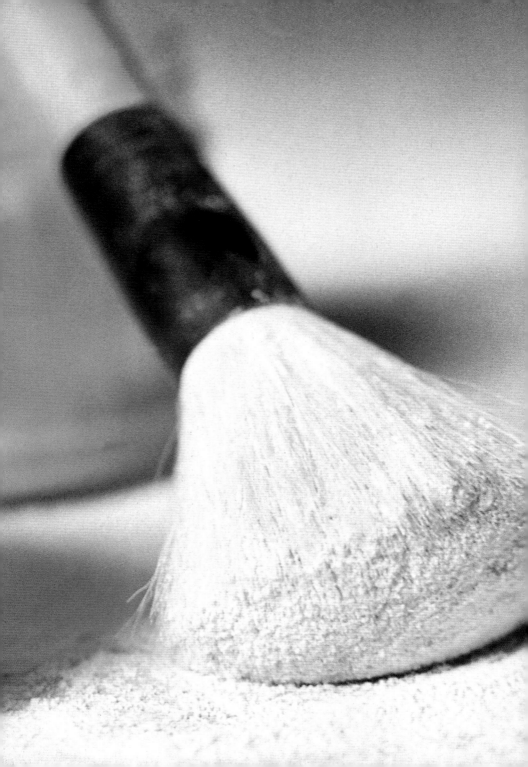

UNDERCOVER

UNDERCOVER

All make-up has the potential to clog your pores. Occasional spots as well as true acne can be brought on by certain cosmetics and toiletries including make-up, foundation, night creams, cleansers and moisturizers. These products often contain mineral oil or petroleum jelly, which can clog pores. Cosmetic acne is less of a problem today because of the vast array of non-comedogenic products on the market. Using the right formula of foundation and powder can absorb oil. Oil-free foundations and concealers are a must-have. They can be a great help with covering up swelling and red spots as they heal, and actually speed up the process. You may find it difficult to apply foundation during the first few weeks of treatment because skin may be red or scaly from the remedies you are using. Waterproof formulas don't come off with soap and water and require more careful cleansing and rubbing to remove. These are not usually recommended for acne-prone skin. The trick is to NEVER go to bed without removing your make-up completely so there is no residue left on the skin overnight.

scar face

Acne scars can present a marathon challenge for make-up gurus when trying to cover effectively because they are generally not flat, but either raised or sunken.

For depressed scars: Fill them in by starting with a primer to allow foundation to flow on smoothly. On top, foundation applied with a sponge gives a flawless finish for recessed areas.

For darkened or red scars: Start with a pale yellow concealer, add a second coat that's a few shades lighter than your skin colour. Top off with concealer that matches your skin tone and set each layer with pressed powder.

Celebrities and their make-up artists know a great deal about the power of good lighting and scar minimizing make-up. When your face is broadcast on multiplex screens all around the globe, even the tiniest defect can get magnified. Without carefully placed concealer and just the right primer and foundation, not every cheek, chin, forehead and neck in Hollywood would be ready for a close-up.

Make-up experts can be brilliant at covering up what they don't want us to see, and stars are living proof that nobody's perfect.

MAKE-UP MUST-HAVE:
powder compact and blotting papers for emergency oil spills.

make-up manoeuvres

- Apply make-up to a face that has been cleansed and is completely dry.

- Only use oil-free foundation. On older or combination skin, you can try a formula with a little oil. Use a small amount applied in five dots. One on the forehead, one on the tip of the nose, one on each cheek and one on the chin.

- Gently pat dots of concealer that matches your skin tone under the eyes, on the lids, on any broken capillaries or on very red, blemished areas. Use a camouflage brush or a cotton swab to blend it in. Green-tinted concealer can help to get the red out. Yellow is preferred for correcting bluish skin discolourations, dark circles under the eyes and pasty complexions.

- Use a fine matte powder all over the face, lids and around the lips to control oil. Choose a shade that won't change the hue of your concealer. Even if you don't use foundation, powder is key.

- If you forget or skip the powder phase, the foundation will mix with the natural oils in your skin and melt during the day.

buffed up

If you suffer from acne, choose your beautician wisely. Not all therapists are trained in the accurate assessment of problem skin and its special needs.

All acne treatments should be given under sanitary conditions to provide the most healing results. Mild steam cleansing coupled with an exfoliation treatment to remove dead topical cells, extractions and a soothing, healing mask is the best course. Facial scrubs that buff away excess oil, dirt and dead skin can also give skin a big boost. However, rubbing and massaging can cause irritation and intense facial massage, rich European-style facial creams and over-handling of delicate pores can aggravate acne and cause eruptions. If your skin looks like it went through a war after a facial treatment, your technician is heavy handed and too aggressive.

Extracting whiteheads

Whiteheads are closed comedos and should only be extracted in the hands of an expert. A dermatologist may use a sterile needle to prick the tip of the pimple – do not try this at home. When you squeeze them yourself, you risk making the situation worse. As an alternative, try applying a salicylic gel or cream to help unplug the pore. Sometimes applying ice to the area whenever you feel the urge to touch it, can help.

DIY acne facial

- **Cleansing:** Apply a cleanser with the fingertips and work into the skin. Remove completely with a face cloth.

- **Steaming:** Apply a warm cloth to the face to soften the skin and relax pores.

- **Extraction:** With a tissue around your two fingers, gently squeeze the pore. If the oil plug isn't released, abort the mission. Using fingertips and a clean, dry cotton pad, gently press around clogged pores to remove surface debris.

- **Astringent:** Wipe the skin clean with a mild alcohol-free toner.to remove any residue.

- **Mask:** Apply a clay-based purifying mask. Leave this on the face for 10 minutes.

- **Spray:** Wipe off the mask with a warm face cloth and follow with a cooling mist to close pores.

TOP TIP:
Don't have a facial too often (more than once every 6 weeks) and don't have a treatment when your skin is flared up.

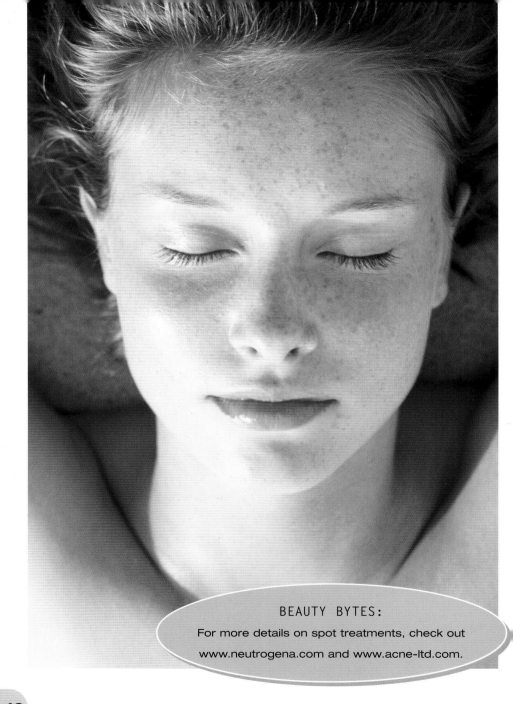

BEAUTY BYTES:

For more details on spot treatments, check out

www.neutrogena.com and www.acne-ltd.com.

sun spots

As many as one third of acne sufferers report that summer is the worst time of year for spots, while some women firmly believe that sun or sun beds dry out and improve their skin

Warmer weather and humidity can bring on breakouts. Sun creams and lotions can clog pores that are open wide from the heat, so they absorb them more readily. Catching rays will not clear up acne. Small amounts of sun exposure may initially make it better, but continuous sunning can increase plugging of the pores that produce blackheads, whiteheads and small spots. A suntan can temporarily dry up some of the oil, but the drying factor could actually encourage the skin to produce more oil. Prolonged exposure to the sun can worsen the condition. Many acne treatments, especially vitamin A derivatives like Isotretinoin and some antibiotics like Doxycycline, increase the skin's sensitivity to ultraviolet light, making the risk of sunburn greater. As a suntan will darken the skin, the lesion will take longer to fade into distant memory. An SPF15 should be used daily for protection, even on spot-prone skin. Without it, instead of spots, you'll have more wrinkles. Sun exposure is a lose, lose situation no matter how you look at it.

body beautiful

Spots are not limited to the oily T-zone of the face. They can show up anywhere, any time. A number of factors including stress and hormones can induce acne lesions on the body.

Acne develops on those areas of the skin where sebaceous glands are most numerous: the face, scalp, neck, chest, back, upper arms and shoulders. Perspiration and snug clothing are two of the most common causes of body acne, which explains why many physically active women are plagued by it. Tight-fitting clothing such as spandex traps perspiration against the skin, allowing it to mix with surface oils. The result is a film that clogs pores and causes blemishes ranging from whiteheads to inflamed papules and pustules. Anyone who sweats through exercise and doesn't properly cleanse their skin afterwards, is only inviting more flare-ups. Sweat traps dirt and oil in the pores, making it very important to shower after any workout. High temperatures and humidity act in the same way, causing sweat to block the pores.

TOP TIP: Never use creamy hair lotions or wear headbands that can clog pores around the hairline and on the back.

If you have oily hair, shampoo daily but avoid heavy conditioners or styling products. If you have breakouts on your forehead, having a fringe may be a contributing factor. Style hair so that it is off your face and neck.

Treatments for body acne are similar to those for the face, but the former is more resistant to treatment because it is harder to reach. We certainly can't see it very well, and we never really know when the pores get congested or we're overdue for emergency exfoliation.

Acne mechanica is a form of acne that is caused by heat, pressure and repetitive frictional rubbing against the skin. It can be the result of wearing tight synthetic sports gear, rucksacks, tight bra straps and underwear. Women with a predisposition to acne on the shoulders, back and buttocks are especially at risk of acne mechanica from wearing equipment straps and clothing. It can be prevented by wearing a clean, cotton T-shirt under sports clothes: cotton absorbs sweat and reduces friction against the skin. Shower immediately after doing any sports, or wash the chest, back and other areas prone to acne. Cleansers containing salicylic acid are good for removing surface oils and unclogging pores. Apply an anti-acne medication like a keratolytic solution to spots as soon as they appear.

TOP TIP:
Peroxide can bleach or stain clothing, so if you are using it for back acne, take this into consideration when choosing what to wear.

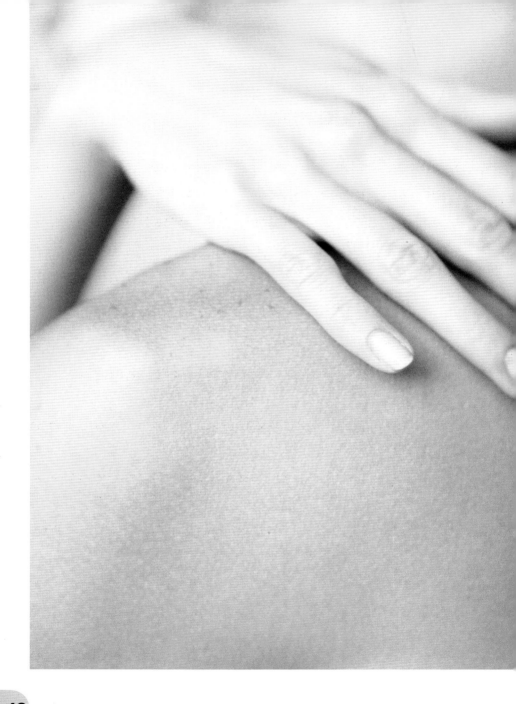

backne regime

What could be worse than spots on your back that show up just when you want to wear a skimpy top? If you're prone to back breakouts, ask your partner or a girlfriend to check out bits you can't get to on your own.

- **DO** pat dry. Don't wipe or rub vigorously as this can irritate.

- **DO** wash twice daily with a salicylic acid based cleanser

- **DO** wipe the affected area with a benzoyl peroxide or salicylic acid pad.

- **DO** follow with an alpha hydroxy acid based body lotion to help exfoliate skin while preventing it from drying out.

- **DO** use a salicylic acid or benzoyl peroxide spot treatment on individual areas at night.

- **DON'T** ever pick or squeeze spots on the back or chest, where the skin is thicker and more prone to scarring.

- **DON'T** forget to shower as soon as possible after perspiring from sports or activity.

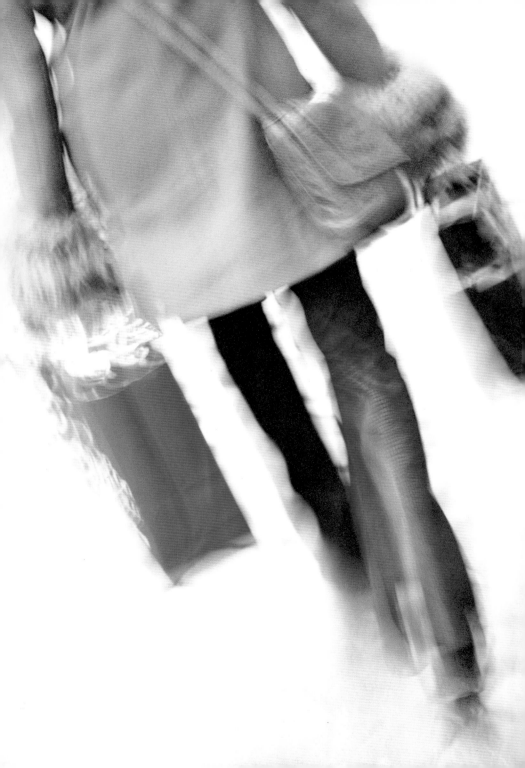

AT THE CHEMIST

Sources of effective and scientific non-prescription treatments have become more important than ever before. Finding a treatment best suited to your needs can take a lot of experimentation. Using too much or the wrong type of formula can give your face a shiny look and clog pores. Acne can't be cured completely, but it can be successfully controlled. Choosing the right products is paramount.

Over-the-counter treatments for mild to moderate acne work by reducing the amount of oil that is produced and by reducing the bacteria that cause infection. Anti-bacterials prevent infection from spreading. Anti-inflammatories reduce swelling, redness and inflammation. Keratolytics normalize the shedding of the follicle lining and remove dead cells.

drying out

Although there is a huge variety of acne treatments on the market, the majority of them contain the same few vital ingredients.

Prescription and over-the-counter benzoyl peroxide work in the same way but prescription formulas have higher concentrations. It is prescribed most often to make sure patients get the best formulation for their type of acne, either a cream, gel or lotion. Benzoyl peroxide kills bacteria and reduces oil production. Salicylic acid, sulfur and resourcinol help dissolve blackheads and whiteheads. Topical medicines such as over-the-counter creams and gels are applied directly to the spotty or spot-prone area. Most of these help to dry out the excess oil and block the spread of infection. For mild acne, doctors often recommend using an over-the-counter remedy before resorting to more serious treatments that require a prescription. Be patient. It may take a month to see results from over-the-counter products.

Benzoyl peroxide – comes in creams, gels and lotions. It destroys the *P. acnes* bacteria by penetrating the follicle and releasing hydrogen peroxide. For more than just a few spots, spread a thin film of cream or ointment over the entire area to prevent the acne from spreading. BP's main drawback is that it can cause irritation, dryness, peeling or redness, and many women stop using it for that reason.

Benzoyl Peroxide
Concentration 2.5, 5, 10
Kills bacteria, removes shedding cells from follicle

Salicylic acid – found in creams, lotions and pads, it fights blackheads and whiteheads. Salicylic acid is a beta hydroxy acid that is oil soluble and can therefore penetrate oil-plugged pores. It works by destroying the plug and shedding the cells lining the follicles. You must use salicylic acid treatments continually in order to reap the benefits, as pores clog up again once you stop.

Salicylic acid
Concentration 0.5, 2
Removes shedding cells from follicle

Sulphur
Concentration 3 - 10
Kills bacteria, removes shedding cells from follicle

Sulphur – in creams and lotions, sulphur acts as a drying agent by reducing bacteria to help unclog pores and control white-heads and inflamed spots.

Sulphur/Resourcinol – can be found in creams and lotions and is usually combined with salicylic acid or benzoyl peroxide to unclog pores.

Sulphur/Resourcinol
Concentration 3 – 10.6
Kills bacteria, removes shedding cells from follicle

Glycolic acid
Concentration up to 10
Removes shedding cells from follicle

Glycolic acid – high potency glycolic acids including beta hydroxy acid and lactic acid are able to remove excess oils and surface debris to unclog pores.

good medicine

When it comes to benzoyl peroxide, the secret is not to overdo it. Follow the tips below to get the most out of your benzoyl peroxide treatment.

- **Start** with a mild strength of 2.5% to test how your skin reacts to it. Apply a thin layer wherever you are likely to get acne, not just directly onto spots. If irritation or severe redness occurs, skip a day.

- **Week 1** – apply the cream or ointment once a day, then wash it off after one hour.

- **Week 2** – leave it on for two hours every evening if no redness or dryness occurs.

- **Week 3** – by the third week, you should be able to leave it on overnight.

Injections

In some cases, isolated cysts can be injected by a doctor, with a mild steroid solution to dissolve them and speed up healing. It's a great quick fix in a beauty emergency. One shot can dissolve the cyst in 12–24 hours. A mild concentration of benzoyl peroxide might be prescribed to destroy the bacteria. If you have too many injections, or too much steroid is used, a slight depression or dent may result.

Benzoyl Peroxide Preparations

Brand Name	Form
Acne-Aid	Cream
Benzac AC	Gel, wash
Brevoxyl	Gel
Clearasil 10%	Lotion
Benoxyl	Gel
Clearasil Maximum strength	Cream
Desquam-E	Gel
Fostex BPO	Gel, cream
Neutrogena Acne Mask	Mask
Noxzema Acne 12	Lotion
Oxy 5, 10	Cream
Pan Oxyl	Gel, soap bar
Persa-Gel	Gel
Triaz	Lotion
Vanoxide	Lotion

This is a partial list to be used as a guide. Not all over-the-counter products are available in all countries, and brand names vary. Some drugs that require a prescription in the UK, are available over the counter in other countries. Check with your doctor or pharmacist to find out what medications are available to you.

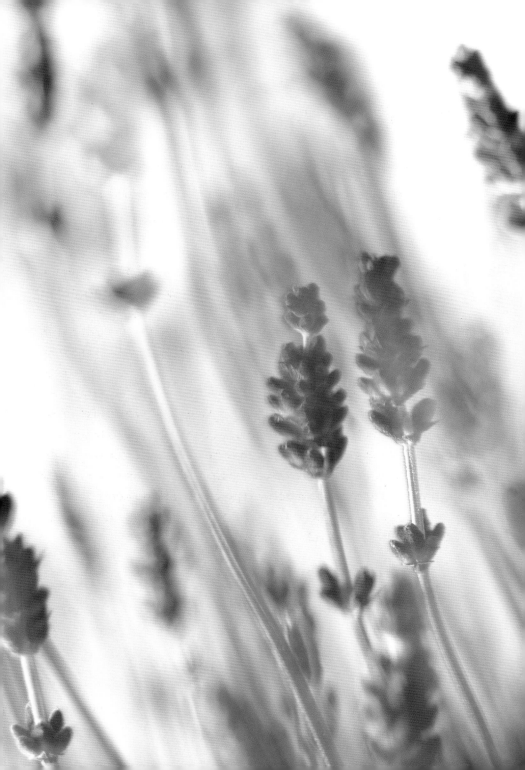

the naturals

If you're determined to go herbal, some natural plant extracts and enzymes can help soothe swelling and mattify the parts of your face with the most oil glands.

The value of alternative medicine for the treatment of acne is up for grabs. Alternative therapies are not medicines prescribed by a doctor, therefore it is difficult to quantify their effectiveness. Before you buy, find out how many people it has helped, if there are any side effects, will it interact with any other medications you are taking and are there potential allergens in it. Even though an ingredient may be completely natural, nothing is ever totally reaction proof. Sensitive skin types can still be irritated by many botanicals. Some alternative preparations may interfere with prescription acne medications, so check with a pharmacist before you take them.

If your skin is super sensitive, you may be wise to try using tea tree oil instead of benzoyl peroxide. A topical solution of 5 per cent tea tree oil has been compared to 5 per cent benzoyl peroxide for mild acne. Tea tree oil works slower, but also has fewer side effects. Topical solutions from 5–15 per cent dilution are available in health food stores.

naturally clear

Naturopaths take a different view from dermatologists when it comes to acne causes and treatments. Several nutritional supplements have been touted to reduce the intensity of acne flare-ups. Responses vary and you'll have to be the judge.

Zinc – reduces inflammation, aids in healing of tissue and preventing scarring and is required for the production of the skin's super antioxidants that reduce the damage of free radicals. Zinc deficiency may trigger acne.
Food sources: whole grain cereals, nuts, seeds and legumes.

Pantothenic acid (vitamin B5) – another of the B complex vitamins that helps prevent and treat some kinds of acne, as well as promote healing of blemishes and reduce sebum production.
Food sources: brewer's yeast, whole-grain breads and cereals, mushrooms, liver, dried beans and peas, avocados, fish, chicken, pecans, hazelnuts, peanuts, cauliflower, milk and cheese, potatoes, oranges, bananas and eggs.

Pyridoxine (vitamin B6) – water-soluble, helps to control outbreaks by regulating levels of hormones implicated in the development of acne lesions.
Food sources: sweet potatoes, avocados, bananas, barley, bok choy, chicken, turkey, potatoes, brown rice, sunflower seeds, tuna, chickpeas, salmon, pork, fresh mangoes.

Topical niacinamide (vitamin B3) – vitamin B3 derivative that penetrates the dermis layer of the skin, stimulating the vasodilation of the blood vessels and increasing blood flow to accelerate the removal of dirt trapped below the skin.
Food sources: peanuts, brewer's yeast, fish, meat, whole grains.

Iron – delivers oxygen from the lungs to all parts of the body, helps the muscles work, and breaks down substances that can damage your body.
Food sources: liver, lean red meat, poultry, fish, oysters, shellfish, kidney, dried beans, fruits, and vegetables.

Linoleic acid – an essential fatty acid that is used as a supplement for hypertension, blood thinning and dermatitis.
Food sources: vegetable oils.

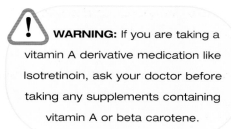

WARNING: If you are taking a vitamin A derivative medication like Isotretinoin, ask your doctor before taking any supplements containing vitamin A or beta carotene.

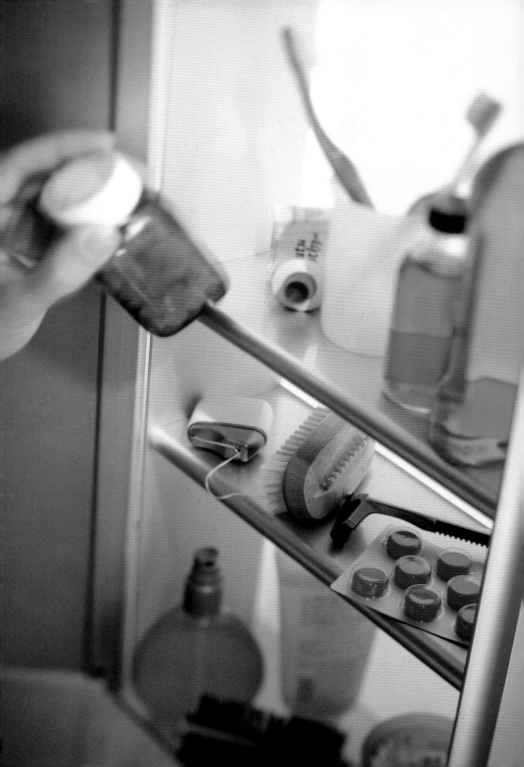

AT THE DOCTOR

You may start by trying to cure acne with home remedies, but
there comes a time when only a doctor will do. With a
dermatologist's help, the good news is that almost every case of
acne can be cleared up, at least temporarily. The products you
get at the local chemist may offer temporary relief from some
forms of acne, but they won't clear up cysts that lie deep within
the skin, or prevent new spots from sprouting up. Some forms of
moderate to severe acne are best treated with prescription
medications, which help to unclog pores and control the acne.

If you have a blemish that won't go away on its own and
doesn't respond to your acne regime, you should see a
dermatologist. Don't let a chronic problem get out of control
without having it checked. A doctor can treat your acne from the
inside out with oral and topical medications. No one should have
to suffer with acne indefinitely when there are safe and
effective medications available. After diagnosing your type of
acne and the severity, your doctor will work with you to
determine a starting point for treatment.

see spot run

When it's time to get serious about spot removal, it's time to look to prescription therapies. These work faster than over-the-counter versions because they are generally more potent.

Like many over-the-counter remedies, most prescription topical medications come in a variety of forms. Your doctor will consider your skin type. Creams and lotions are moisturizing and tend to be good for people with dry skin. Gels and solutions are generally alcohol based and tend to dry out the skin. They work best if you have excessively oily skin or live in a hot, humid climate. All forms work to reduce sebum production, ease inflammation, kill bacteria and stabilize the androgen level. For acne breakouts in harder to reach areas like the back or shoulders, oral medication may be easier to use than topical antibiotics. Topical vitamin A derivatives are considered the cornerstone of an anti-acne treatment plan, and Retin-A® is still odds on favourite among dermatologists.

The biggest mistake that women make is waiting it out. Avoiding treatment can make your spot condition worse and increase your chances of scarring. You can kick your pimple habit, and the earlier you begin, the better. Most topical acne medications should be used on all acne-prone areas including the forehead, cheeks, chin and nose, not just individual spots. Part of the goal is to treat the skin before eruptions begin, and not only to treat the ones you already have. Remember to stay on the prescribed therapy until your doctor says otherwise. It took a while for the pimples to develop, so don't expect them to disappear overnight, even with medical treatment. Most treatments take two to eight weeks before significant results are noticeable. If you haven't seen positive results after two months of taking your medication as directed, or if you've been on the same medication for a year and you're still breaking out, speak to your doctor about changing your medication.

in the clear

Antibiotics are the most common place to start to treat mild to moderate cases of acne.

Antibiotics – In a capsule form, antibiotics are often used together with other therapies. The antibiotic works to destroy *p. acnes* bacteria to reduce inflammation, redness and pus formation. In many cases, you will need to stay on oral antibiotics for 2 to 4 months at a time. You should finish the course unless otherwise directed by your doctor. If it is interrupted, they may become ineffective. You must follow your doctor's directions for how to take your medication, to the letter. Some antibiotics should be taken on an empty stomach. Some are more effective when they are taken with or after meals. You might be told to take them at least one hour before bedtime. Your doctor may advise you not to take other medications or supplements – like iron or calcium – while taking some antibiotics, because they can interfere with absorption. Certain types, like the tetracyclines, are harder on the digestive tract, while others are more slowly absorbed and may have fewer side effects. If you are having trouble using the antibiotic prescribed, speak to your doctor about changing your medication. If your acne is coming back even while you are on antibiotics that were previously helpful, you may have become resistant to them. Your doctor may want to switch you to a different class of antibiotics. Cream, lotion and gel formulas are also commonly used in addition to pills as anti-bacterial agents.

Side effects: Nausea or diarrhoea, sun sensitivity, yeast infections, headache, dizziness, skin discolouration, tooth discolouration.

Oral antibiotics

Drug Class	Brand Name
Tetracycline	Tetracycline, Achromycin, Sumycin
Doxycycline	Doryx, Vibramycin
Minocycline	Dynacin, Minocin, Vectrin
Erythromycin	E-mycin, Ery-C, Ery-tab, E.E.S., Ery-ped, Erthrocin, PCE
Penicillin-type drugs	Ampicillin, Cephalexin
Sulfa	Bactrim, Cotrim, Septra

This is a partial list to be used as a guide. Not all drugs are available in all countries and generic and brand names vary. Some medications that require a prescription in the UK, are available over the counter in other countries. Check with your doctor or pharmacist to find out what medications are available to you.

Hormonal therapy – The use of birth control pills is common to reduce the amount of androgens in a woman's body. Low-dose corticosteroid drugs, such as Prednisone or Dexamethasone, may have an anti-inflammatory effect and suppress the androgen produced by the adrenal glands. Anti-androgen drugs, such as Spironolactone, may be prescribed to help prevent androgens from causing excessive oil production.

Side effects: menstrual irregularities, breast tenderness, headache, fatigue.

the A list

Retinoids are derivatives of Vitamin A that work to unclog pores. Retin-A® has been on the market since the 1970s and is commonly used to treat wrinkles, psoriasis and acne.

Retinoids – Most effective in treating blackheads and whiteheads, retinoids also fight acne by increasing cell turnover, which helps unplug existing comedos, so other topical medications, such as antibiotics, can penetrate the follicles better. In the UK and the US, a prescription is required. In other countries, prescription strength retinoids can be found in a pharmacy. One of the downsides is that retinoids can dry out the skin and cause peeling and irritation. Occasionally, the acne worsens during the first month of treatment because the medication draws out spots that would not otherwise have shown up yet. These side effects usually decrease or go away when the medication has been used for a period of time and your skin is used to it. Many women worry that Retin-A® will 'thin the skin'. That is precisely the point. Tretinoin causes a thinning of the epidermis, or outer layer of skin. It is an exfoliating agent or keratolytic, which makes it effective in removing the oil plugs that cause acne blemishes.

How to use retinoids:
Wait 20–30 minutes after cleansing to apply. Apply sparingly and at night. A pea-sized dab is enough for your entire face. Apply sunscreen before going out.

Topical acne drugs

Types of drug	Brand Name	Format
Tazarotene	Tazorac	Cream, gel
Thromycin	ATS	Solution, gel
Erythromycin	Erycette	Pads
	Erygel	Gel
	Erymax	Solution
	Staticin	Solution
	T-Stat	Cream
Clindamycin Phosphate	Cleocin T	Solution, gel, pads
Sulfacetamide	Klaron	Lotion
Sulfur	Sulfacet-R	Lotion
Metronidazole	Metrogel	Gel, cream, lotion
Adapalene	Differin	Gel, pads, cream
Tretinoin	Retin-A	Cream, gel, lotion
	Retin-A Micro	Gel
	Avita	Cream, gel
Azelaic Acid	Azelex	Cream

This is a partial list to be used as a guide. Not all drugs are available in all countries and generic and brand names vary. Some medications that require a prescription in the UK, are available over the counter in other countries. Check with your doctor or pharmacist to find out what medications are available to you.

the last resort

Isotretinoin is used as a last resort to clear up severe cystic acne. Now on the market for over 20 years, Isotretinoin has been shown to be effective for 70–85 per cent of patients.

It comes in 10, 20 or 40mg capsules that are taken with food once or twice daily. In the EC and Canada, topical forms may also be available. The average treatment period is 4 months and the strength and frequency is determined by your doctor.

Additional treatment courses can be given for recurrences. The most likely candidate for repeat treatments is suffering from deep, painful, cystic acne that has not responded to the usual alternatives.

Isotretinoin is currently the only medication that actually shrinks the gland that produces the oily sebum found in acne. It is a potent drug that often produces dramatic results, but it also comes with some serious side effects and potentially life threatening risks. Among the more serious of these are elevated blood cholesterol, lipid and triglyceride levels and abnormal liver enzymes. The side effects you may experience usually go away after the medication is stopped.

BEAUTY BYTES:

For important information about Isotretinoin, log on to www.facefacts.com.

TOP TIP:

Always carry a moisturizing lip balm with shea butter or aloe vera if you are on Isotretinoin, to reapply during the day and prevent lips from cracking.

Careful screening and evaluation will be done before you can start taking the drug, as well as close monitoring and frequent blood tests during therapy. If you have difficulty tolerating it, your doctor may be able to reduce the dose of the drug so that the side effects are reduced or stopped. You will be instructed not to take vitamin A derivatives while you are using this medicine and to avoid the sun. Isotretinoin is expensive if you are paying out of your own pocket.

If you are using ANY form of retinoid therapy, there is increased sensitivity to the sun since the epidermis is thinner, so sunscreen with a minimum SPF 15 is a must. Sun exposure can cause severe irritation or burning and lead to hyperpigmentation and possible scarring.

Side effects: Dry eyes, dry mouth, dry skin, cracked, peeling lips, Itching, nosebleeds, muscle aches.

WARNING: Don't even think about getting pregnant while taking Isotretinoin. This drug cannot be taken during pregnancy or while breastfeeding because it can cause severe birth defects.

peels

Chemical peels are used to unroof pustules and exfoliate the skin. Exfoliation helps topical treatments to penetrate the skin in order to control acne and prevent further outbreaks.

Peeling principles are based on the fact that the cells in the epidermis regenerate every month. Peels cause a burn in the skin similar to sunburn, depending upon the type of compound used and its concentration. The top layers of skin – epidermis and dermis – are scraped off. 24 hours after the procedure, new skin cells begin to form a new top layer. 1 to 2 days later, more new cells called fibroblastic cells become active in the dermis. These cells create new collagen fibres, which constitute the support structure of the newly generated skin. At the same time, the elastin fibres, which give the skin its flexibility, also begin to regenerate. Peels of sufficient depth can produce inflammation, redness of the skin and swelling. Peeling agents that reach the under-layers of the skin cause some degree of injury, and then, actually peel some of the cells in the epidermis.

Most superficial to moderate peels are performed in the doctor's surgery and the procedure takes about 30 minutes. It begins with deep skin cleansing, after which the peeling compound is applied. This remains on the skin for a few minutes, causing burning and stinging. Lighter peels are typically repeated at intervals of 3–4 weeks, until the desired effect is achieved. A monthly or bi-monthly maintenance programme will help keep acne under control and between treatments, creams that contain retinoic or glycolic acid should be used regularly, to preserve the results of the

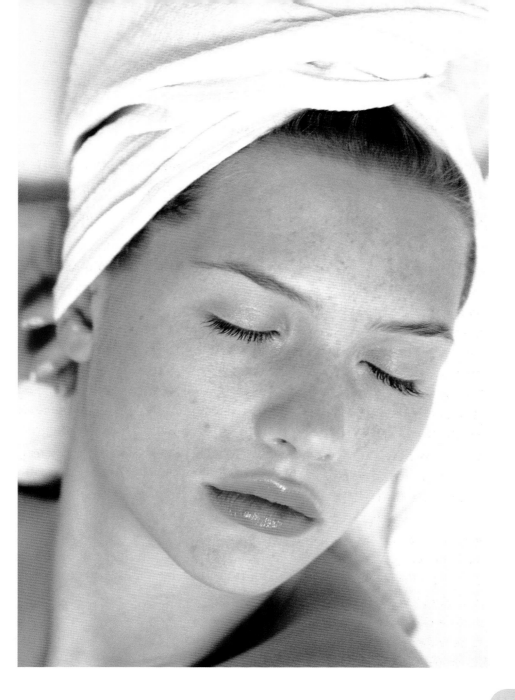

treatment. One significant advantage of superficial peels as opposed to medium or deep peels is that the change is not as drastic and the results will not draw undue attention. Superficial or 'lunchtime' peeling revitalizes the outer layers of skin, for a smooth, rejuvenated appearance. Medium depth peeling is usually recommended for fair-skinned individuals, but superficial face peels can be done on darker skinned patients without the danger of new dark spots appearing. For acne, peeling can considerably reduce the number of blemishes and can improve skin colour, transforming it from yellowish and dull to pink and smooth.

Alpha hydroxy Acid (AHA) – superficial glycolic peels can be repeated as needed, to exfoliate and keep pores open and clean. Daily use of a peel with a glycolic acid based lotion will contribute to continued clearing of the skin.

Beta hydroxy Acid (BHA) – salicylic acid, the ingredient in aspirin, is often used to treat acne because it reduces inflammation as well as blackheads and spots. Salicylic acid is oil soluble and can therefore penetrate oil plugged pores.

Trichloracetic acid (TCA) – a deeper peel that penetrates into the dermis. TCA peels work well to lighten pigmented acne scars and even out skin tone. A TCA peel is usually done once every few months. Deeper TCA peels produce burning, redness and peeling that are more severe, and may take a week or more to heal.

Peel Alternatives

Micro dermabrasion – a state-of-the-art peel that produces no downtime. The treatment uses a high-powered combination of force plus suction to deliver finely ground aluminium oxide or sodium crystals to give the skin a remarkably smooth texture. It can reduce acne and related scarring, enlarged pores and surface lesions, and forestall breakouts.

let there be light

Moving beyond the pharmacy, new light-based therapies may offer the next wave in acne treatments. In theory, these could cause less irritation than traditional drug therapies.

One new technology emits a narrow band spectrum of intense violet-blue light to destroy bacteria found in acne. When the high intensity lamp is shined directly on the skin, it kills the bacteria. Devices like the ClearLight™ may be able to achieve better results than antibiotics and destroy acne-causing bacteria for a few months. Another system uses a green wavelength of heat and light over the face and body to clear acne. The ClearTouch Acne Clearance System stimulates the body's natural defences against acne by producing oxygen. A typical plan will include treatments twice a week for 4 weeks, followed by a maintenance programme. Studies indicate that in 3 or 4 weeks as much as 60–70 per cent of the lesions can be healed. Topical medications can be used in conjunction with light therapy when needed. Clinical studies are also underway to evaluate the effectiveness of laser systems like the N-Lite® in treating active acne. The future looks bright.

BEAUTY BYTES:

For more information about light therapy, log on to www.acneworld.com.

wrinkles and acne

As if puberty wasn't tough enough, what do you do when you can't decide whether your wrinkles or your spots are your biggest skin care concern?

You've got crow's-feet and frown lines, as well as spots on your cheeks, chin and forehead. While the demand for anti-wrinkle products increases steadily, women have an insatiable appetite for new and improved acne therapies.

Skin has a pH balance of 5.5. If you're mistreating your skin by using harsh detergents, over-cleansing, over-scrubbing or layering on acids, your pH may climb to 7.5 or higher. Healthy skin will bounce back quickly, but if your skin is under siege it can take longer to recover, leaving it more susceptible to stress. A normal pH of 5.5 protects skin from bacteria, which tend to thrive in a more alkaline environment. It is important to keep the skin moisturized while treating the breakouts. The areas of the face that contain the fewest oil glands, like around the eyes and the neck, need hydration. Using a non-comedogenic moisturizer is key for dry areas.

For mature skins suffering from lines and lesions, the name of the game is gentle exfoliation. In these cases, mild forms of vitamin A like a low dose of prescription-strength tretinoin or over-the-counter retinoids, are ideal. They can work within the skin's surface where wrinkles start. Combined with a gentle formula of alpha and beta hydroxy acids, you can keep pores clean and prevent future breakouts.

darker skin

*Dark skin is prone to post inflammatory hyperpigmentation –
a darkening or discolouring that occurs after an acne lesion
has healed or when a treatment has caused inflammation.*

The darker your skin, the darker the hyperpigmentation is likely to be and
the longer it will take to lighten. Bleaching dark spots takes months so be
patient. Lightening treatments must be used consistently to work. Black
skin is prone to scarring and dark blotches. It discolours quickly. Asian skin
has yellow undertones and is transparent and soft, meaning it magnifies
every mark. Latin skin is firm, tough and generally oilier than other types.

A Day at the Bleach

Only apply bleaching agent to affected areas as it will lighten any skin it
touches. Apply it to clean, dry skin. Wait 20 minutes before using any other
creams. UV protection is vital as the sun will work against the bleach. Stop
the treatment when the area has lightened up sufficiently. Hydroquinone is
the most effective skin lightening ingredient but not everyone can tolerate
it. Kojic Acid works well for darker skin
types. Glycolic acids can help the
bleaching agent to penetrate
the skin better.

BEAUTY BYTES:
For info on ethnic skin care, go to
www.skinsite.com, www.black-net.com and
www.ethnicbeautyonline.com.

questions

questions

Keep a journal of your acne history; what worked and what didn't, when your acne seems to flare up and potential causes. A dermatologist will evaluate the severity of your acne and suggest the therapy that they have had the most success with in treating other cases similar to yours.

Questions you should ask your doctor:

- Are there better medications to clear up my acne than the ones I've tried?

- How long will it take for my acne to clear up?

- How often should I wash the affected area?

- What is the next step if this method doesn't work effectively?

- What is the best combination of medications for my type of acne?

- What cosmetic and skin care ingredients should I avoid?

- Should I avoid certain foods?

- What else can I do to help clear up my acne?

Questions your doctor might ask you:

- How long have you had acne?

- What skin products are you now using and have you used in the past?

- What medications are you currently taking?

- When do flare-ups most often occur?

- In what areas on your body and face do you have blemishes?

- Have you seen other doctors about it before?

- What treatments have you already tried?

- Did any of the treatments work? If so, which ones?

- Did your parents have acne when they were young?

- If so, how bad was their acne?

- Do you have a history of any hormonal imbalances?

- If so, what are your symptoms?

- How active are you and how much sun exposure do you get?

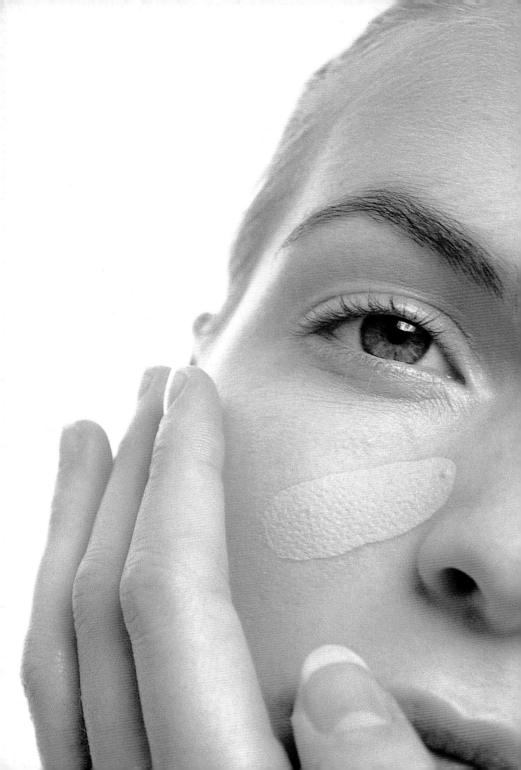

SCAR WARS

SCAR WARS

Old acne scars from your turbulent teens can ruin an otherwise smooth complexion at any age. The best way to prevent scars is to treat acne early, and for as long as is necessary. If left untreated, acne can cause significant scarring later on. Scars are the visible reminders of injury and tissue repair. In the case of acne, the injury is caused by the body's inflammatory response to sebum, bacteria and dead cells in the plugged follicle.

Some people scar more easily than others and it varies from one person to the next. This marking of the skin frequently results from severe inflammatory cystic acne that occurs deep in the skin, and can also arise from more superficial spots. Some women bear their acne scars for a lifetime and notice little change in them. In others, the skin undergoes some degree of remodelling and blemishes diminish in size. It is difficult to predict who will scar, how extensive or deep scars will be, how long they will persist and how successfully scars can be prevented by effective treatment. The more inflammation can be prevented, the more likely it is that scarring can be avoided.

leaving a mark

Acne commonly leads to the formation of depressed or pitted scarring due to inflammation affecting the dermal layer of the skin.

Pseudo Scars

Macules are the flat, red or reddish spots that are the final stage of most inflamed acne lesions. After a spot heals, a macule may remain for 6–12 months or longer depending on skin type. Post-inflammatory pigmentation, the discolouration of the skin at the site of a healed spot, occurs more frequently in darker-skin types, but can also be seen in lighter skin. Excessive sun exposure can cause a healing spot to darken and thus, take longer to fade. These scars change from bluish to ivory white in colour in light skinned people, and become much less obvious.

Depressed Scars

Ice pick or chicken pox scars are caused by a loss of tissue and are more common than keloids and hypertrophic scars. They usually occur on the cheek as small dents with a jagged edge and steep sides. They may be

BEAUTY BYTES:

For more info on acne scar treatments, log on to www.stopspots.org.

be shallow or deep, and hard or soft to the touch. Soft scars can be improved by stretching the skin; hard scars cannot be stretched out. Depressed fibrotic scars are usually deeper and larger. If blemishes are really deep on a woman in her 40s, a facelift procedure may smooth out the skin in the process.

Raised scars

Keloids or hypertrophic scars are caused by an overgrowth of scar tissue. Overproduction of collagen is a response of skin cells to injury and the excess collagen becomes piled up in fibrous masses, which leaves a firm, irregularly shaped scar. They are typically 1 to 2 mm in diameter, but some may be over 1 cm. Occasionally they can be injected with a mild steroid to shrink the scar. Keloid scars tend to run in families, and are more common on the upper body and in darker skin types.

Superficial scars

These are commonly clusters of lone shallow scars that can show up on the forehead, cheek and chin areas. They are not usually deep enough to be filled and are best levelled with multiple peeling or resurfacing treatments.

scar remedies

Total restoration of the skin to the way it looked before acne first attacked is not usually possible, but everything can be improved to some extent.

The most common souvenir is uneven skin texture, especially visible on the softer areas of the face like the cheeks. This is caused by tough scar tissue that forms both on the surface and in the deeper skin layers. Acne erupts from the deep tissue to the surface of the skin, so the scars it leaves behind can be more complex than those from cuts and scrapes. Acne scars are three-dimensional because they go through the skin.

Acne scar fillers

Form	Brand Name
Bovine collagen	Zyplast®, Zyderm®
Bovine collagen with micro particles	ArteColl®
Human tissue	Fat, Cymetra® Fascian®
Hyaluronic acid	Restylane®, Perlane®, Hylaform®
Injectable liquid silicone	Silskin®
Hyaluronic acid with acrylic hydrogel fragments	Dermalive®

Fillers

For depressed scars, fillers such as your own fat, collagen and hyaluronic acid gel can be injected under the skin to stretch and fill out certain types of soft scars. Human collagen or fascia (the tissue covering the muscles) can also be used. Fat is taken from another site on your own body and injected beneath the surface of the skin to elevate depressed scars. In almost all cases, fillers will have to be repeated.

Resurfacers

Many of the treatments that are used to keep acne under control, are also helpful in taking care of the scars it leaves behind, only in a deeper mode.

Microdermabrasion – uses aluminium oxide crystals passing through a vacuum tube to remove surface skin and smooth down ridges. Multiple procedures, often deeper than the customary treatments, will be needed to soften acne scarring.

Dermabrasion – involves using a high-speed brush to remove surface skin and alter the contour of deeper scars. In darker-skinned people, dermabrasion may cause changes in pigmentation that require additional treatment.

Chemical peels – a series of glycolic acid, beta hydroxy acid and trichloracetic acid peels (TCA) can be used in varying strengths to improve the appearance of scars left from acne lesions.

Ablative Laser Treatments

Lasers of various wavelength and intensities are used to recontour scar tissue and reduce the redness around healed acne lesions. Ablative laser technologies can improve the deepest scars that remain decades after acne has run its course, and in some cases, a single treatment will achieve permanent results. The downside is that because the skin absorbs bursts of energy from the laser, there may be post-treatment redness for several months. The CO_2 laser vaporizes thin layers of the skin and tightens collagen fibres, which is good for depressed acne scars. The Erbium:YAG laser produces very precise bursts of energy, which allows for the sculpting of smaller, irregular scars. CO_2 laser treated sites heal in 7–10 days, while skin treated with the Erbium:YAG laser heals in 5–7 days. Coblation, which uses low-energy frequency to treat scars, falls somewhere between CO_2 and Erbium lasers. It can be used to produce some results on deeper scars with less of a healing period than CO_2, and is generally better than the lighter non-ablatives.

Non-ablative Lasers

Non-ablative lasers are showing promise in softening acne scars but they work slower. The cooling infrared lasers like CoolTouch® cause mild redness for a few hours after the procedure, but no pain. The treatment feels like a rubber band lightly snapping against the skin with an alternating cool and warm sensation. An average of 4 treatments is required to reduce most acne scars and they should be continued monthly as needed. The laser stimulates the body to produce more collagen under the skin. The deeper the scar, the more collagen you have to make to raise the scar up. Less intense lasers don't give immediate results because the collagen takes months to form. Intense Pulsed Light sources and Pulse Dye lasers offer quick treatment alternatives without the downtime, but they must be done in a series to improve scarring. For scars that have turned white over time, the Excimer laser has proved effective in re-pigmenting scar tissue, which is particularly useful for darker skin types more prone to hyperpigmentation (skin discolouring). Combination therapy with a series of laser or light-based treatments and mechanical resurfacing like microdermabrasion can be effective on large, soft areas of the face with rolling scar tissue. The light from a sub-surfacing laser is used to stimulate new collagen growth in the deeper layers of the skin, which can plump out any depressions left from scars.

Skin surgery

Some individual scars may be removed by a punch excision. The scar is excised down to the layer of fat underneath the skin; the resulting hole in the skin may be repaired with sutures or with a small skin graft. 'Subcision' is a technique in which a surgical probe is used to lift the scar tissue away from unscarred skin, to elevate the depressed scar.

TOP TIP:

Often, the best remedy for acne scars is a series of treatments, or a combination of several different ones.

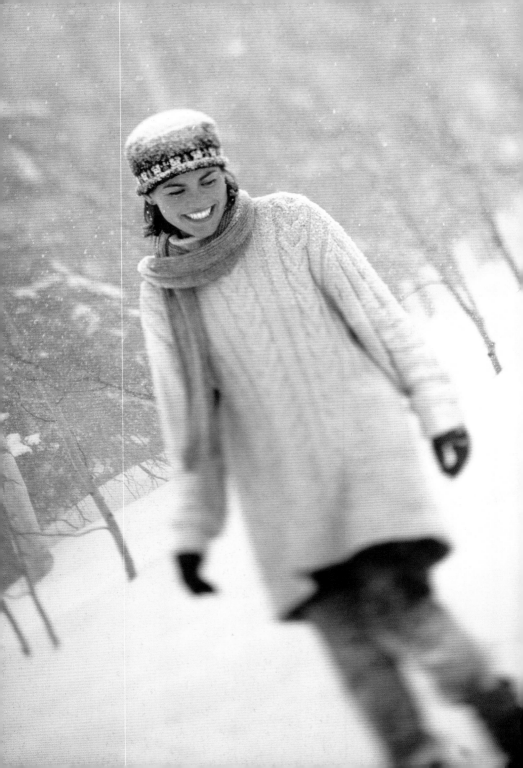

BLUSHING BEAUTY

BLUSHING BEAUTY

There is a definite distinction between garden variety 'acne' or 'acne vulgaris' and 'acne rosacea'. Rosacea and acne are different conditions and require specific treatments. Not every skin eruption or pink blemish is necessarily a telltale sign of acne. For example, milia (small white cysts) on the forehead and back could be sweat bumps. Patchy red spots may be an indication of eczema. True acne is black and white; comedos and pustules that is. Redness or inflammation is generally localized to the acne lesions, and facial veins are not prominent. Rosacea is characterized by a different set of symptoms that includes flushing, broken capillaries and only occasional acne-like skin eruptions that may ooze or crust in the central part of the face. Blackheads and whiteheads are not present. Rosacea's inflammation and redness is vascular in nature. Danger signs include facial redness, flushing, swelling, papules and pustules, dermatitis, stinging, burning, broken blood vessels and bloodshot eyes.

operation avoidance

There is a definite distinction between rosacea and better known types of sensitive skin, although if you have rosacea, your skin might be sensitive to certain things.

Conquering rosacea usually means avoiding anything that may bring on an attack. Culprits vary from person to person. Wash thoroughly with a soap free cleanser and lukewarm water to prevent fungal infections: rosacea medications kill bacteria, creating new space for fungi to grow. Be sensible about what you put on your face in terms of skin care and make-up.

Operation Avoidance

Lifestyle	• Sun exposure (public enemy #1) • Cold and wind • Saunas, hot tubs, steamy showers • Getting overheated • Coughing or straining • Loofahs, sponges, washcloths, abrasives • Smoking
Skin Care Ingredients	• Alcohol • Fragrance • Menthol • Witch-hazel • Peppermint oil • Detergents • Acids • Chemical sunscreens • Astringents
Diet	• Very hot caffeinated drinks (tea, coffee, hot chocolate) • Foods high in niacin (liver, yeast) • Foods containing histamine (tomatoes, aubergine, cheese) • Spices (paprika, chilli, cayenne, oriental mustard) • Alcoholic beverages (wine, beer, spirits)

spotting rosacea

Your face flushes unexpectedly, the broken blood vessels on your cheeks get red and swollen, you get flare-ups of bumps or pimples and sometimes a stinging or burning.

These symptoms may last for hours or days and start up without warning. The bad news is that it sounds like rosacea, a chronic skin condition that has no cure. The good news is that rosacea can be treated, and should be. If left untreated, it will usually get worse. Rosacea is generally diagnosed by what stage it is in; first (mild), second (moderate) or third (severe). It starts later in life than acne and affects the cheeks, chin, nose and forehead. No cause has been definitively linked with rosacea, which makes it difficult to figure out. It is considered a vascular disorder and can be brought on by menopause, high blood pressure, stress or fever. Like most other skin afflictions, it is more common in women than in men. At least 25 per cent of women in their 30s and 40s have rosacea. Statistics indicate that rosacea now ranks as the fifth most common diagnosis made by dermatologists, and it is still considered widely underdiagnosed. People most prone to rosacea are aged between 30 and 60, of Irish, English or Scottish descent, or with northern or eastern European origins, fair skinned, with a family history of rosacea. Having had an adverse reaction to an acne medication or a sty may also be indications.

get the red out

Rosacea is basically a vascular problem, which is why you may appear red in certain places. The skin is thin, so it reveals the redness of the veins that lie right underneath.

Light glycolic acid peels are often used in conjunction with antibiotics to control rosacea. A series of peels are performed every 2–4 weeks along with a skin care programme with a low concentration of glycolic acid washes and creams. The peeled facial skin will be red for a few hours following the treatment, and make-up should be avoided. Tiny facial veins called 'telangiectasias' can be effectively zapped with lasers that emit specific wavelengths of light that target the visible blood vessels just under the skin. Heat from the laser's energy builds in the vessels, causing them to collapse. More than one treatment may be needed, and with the most advanced lasers and laser light devices, there is little or no bruising. Once you've zapped the existing blood vessels, you will need additional treatments for new ones as they crop up. Lasers also work for rhinophyma, a severe stage of rosacea that causes the tip of the nose to swell and the skin to become thickened and bulbous. Fortunately for women, this is much more common in men.

BEAUTY BYTES:
If you think you have rosacea, check out www.rosacea.org and www.acne-rosacea.co.uk.

drug therapies

Many drugs can make rosacea worse, while others can control it. Long-term maintenance treatment is often offered.

Vasodilator drugs, used to dilate the blood vessels, can worsen the condition. Prolonged use of topical steroids or use of topical cortisone of greater than 1 per cent, have been found to aggravate rosacea.

Metronidazole – an antibiotic used topically to treat the inflammation, pustule formation and redness. A thin film is usually applied twice daily in the morning and evening. It may take three weeks or more to see the effects.

Retinoids

Drug	Brand Name
Metronidazole topical	Metrogel, Metrolotion, Metrocream, Noritate
Tretinoin	Differin, Retin-A
Isotretinoin	Accutane, Roaccutane

Not all drugs are available in all countries and generic and brand names vary. Some medications that require a prescription in the UK, are available over the counter in other countries. Check with your doctor or pharmacist to find out what medications are available to you.

rosacea diary

rosacea diary

To help isolate the factors that cause rosacea to flare up, keep a daily diary of your activities and the foods and substances you come into contact with.

TODAY'S DATE

Weather conditions

Sunny	Hot	Cold	Humid	Windy

What you consumed today

Spicy foods

Alcohol

Hot beverages

Fruits

Dairy products

Vegetables

Medications

Other

What happened today

Emotional stress

Physical exertion

Hot bath/sauna

Warm room temperatures

Symptoms

List the substances you came into contact with today

Skin care products

Cosmetics

Soap

Perfume

Aftershave

Shampoo

Household products

Other

What is the condition of your rosacea today?

No flare-up   Mild flare-up   Severe flare-up

SUMMING IT UP

SUMMING IT UP

While there is still no permanent cure for acne, there are many treatments that can control the sequence of events that cause it. Acne occurs when sebaceous hair follicles trap the oily substance they produce, called sebum. It can be caused by changes in hormone levels, stress and certain environmental or genetic factors. The arsenal of effective acne treatments includes antibacterial creams, lotions or gels including benzoyl peroxide, that can be used alone or in combination with topical or oral antibiotics such as erythromycin or clindamycin. Anti-inflammatory medications called corticosteroids may be injected directly into severe inflamed acne lesions to help clear them up. Topicals such as Retin-A®, Azelex® and Tazorac® help unclog oil ducts. Certain low-dose birth control pills may also help to clear the skin. For severe cystic acne, Roaccutane (Accutane) is usually the answer. Treatment has to be tailored to suit your individual case of acne. Some women's complexions are very oily, so they need drying topical agents, others may need mild medication because their skin is dry and some women have oily skin in the centre of the face and dry areas on the sides. That's why a lot of women get into trouble with over-the-counter products. Start with a glycolic acid or salicylic acid cleanser from a chemist. If your skin gets dry, use oil-free moisturizer straight away.

If your skin does not get too dry or irritated, use a benzoyl peroxide product and then try a glycolic acid cream to clear out your pores at night. If you find that you are not responding to over-the-counter remedies, see a dermatologist to have treatment tailored to your needs.

Many new treatments are on the market today to help heal acne and even reduce the scarring. If your first attempts at achieving acne-free skin are unsuccessful, there will always be other avenues to explore. As skin is unique to the individual, medication that works wonders for your best friend may not be the thing for you. However, every treatment will work to some extent for some women. Finding what works is a constantly evolving process. You have to be proactive in keeping up with new developments, changing your regime or seeking medical help, as your acne will go through stages. Studies point to combination therapy to maximize effectiveness, minimize inflammation that can lead to scarring and control flare-ups. Be patient. Most treatments take 4–8 weeks to start working. Women with acne want an instant cure, but there isn't one. The best you can hope for is a gradual improvement. The good news is that the variety of treatments is expanding and improving all the time, so even for women who have carried visible reminders of their acne for many years, there is always hope.

index

acids, 31
acne mechanica, 45
acne treatments:
    dermatologists, 59–75
    facials, 40–1
    over-the-counter, 49–57
adapalene, 65
adrenal glands, 63
adult acne, 16–17
alcohols, 31
allergies, 23
alpha hydroxy acid, 70, 72
alternative therapies, 55
anabolic steroids, 13
androgens, 9, 12–13, 63
anti-acne products, 28–9
anti-bacterials, 49
anti-inflammatories, 49
antibiotics, 21, 43, 62–3, 89
astringents, 24, 41
azelaic acid, 65

bacteria, 13, 34, 49, 71
benzoyl peroxide, 21, 45, 50,
    52–3, 55
beta carotene, 57
beta hydroxy acid, 70, 72, 81
birth control pills, 18–19, 63
blackheads, 10, 34
bleaching agents, 73
blood vessels, rosacea, 85–91
body acne, 44–7
bovine collagen, 80

calcium, 62
chemical peels, 68–70, 81, 88

cleansers, 24, 26, 41
clindamycin phosphate, 65
closed comedos, 10
clothing, 44, 45
collagen, 79, 80, 81, 82
comedos, 10, 34
concealer, 35, 37, 38, 39
contraceptive pill, 18–19, 63
corticosteroids, 13, 63
cortisone, 89
cosmetics, 28–31, 37–9
cysts, 11, 34, 52

dark skin, 73
dehydrated skin, 26
depressed scars, 38, 78–9
dermabrasion, 81
dermatologists, 40, 59–75
detergents, 31
Dexamethasone, 63
diet, 23, 56–7, 86
doctors, 59–75
doxycycline, 43, 63
drugs: causing acne, 13
    in pregnancy, 21
    prescription drugs, 60–7
    and rosacea, 89
dry skin, 24, 26

eczema, 85
erythromycin, 63, 65
esters, 31
ethers, 31
exercise, 44, 45
exfoliation, 24, 30, 40, 68, 72
extracting whiteheads, 40, 41

facials, 40–1
fillers, depressed scars, 80–1
follicles, 10, 11, 12–13, 49
food, 23, 56–7, 86
foundation, 37, 38, 39

glycolic acid, 21, 51, 70, 73, 81, 88
glycols, 31
grading acne, 14–15

hair care products, 29, 44
hair styles, 44
herbal remedies, 31, 55
hormones, 9, 12–13, 18–19, 63
hyaluronic acid, 80
hydroquinone, 73
hyperpigmentation, 35, 73, 83
hypertrophic scars, 79

ice pick scars, 78
inflammatory acne, 10, 11
injectable liquid silicone, 80
injections, steroid, 52
iodine, 23
iron, 57, 62
Isotretinoin, 11, 43, 57, 66–7, 89

keloids, 79
keratolytics, 45, 49
Kojic acid, 73

lanolin, 31
laser treatments, 82–3, 88
light-based therapies, 71, 82–3
linoleic acid, 57
macules, 78

make-up, 37–9
masks, 30, 41
mature skin, 72
menopause, 12
menstrual cycle, 18
metronidazole, 65, 89
microdermabrasion, 70, 81, 83
microcomedos, 34
milia, 85
minocycline, 63
moisturizers, 28, 30, 72

naturopathy, 56–7
niacinamide, 57

oestrogen, 18
oils, in skin care products, 31
oily skin, 16, 26
open comedos, 10
oral contraceptives, 18–19, 63
Ortho Tri-Cyclen®, 18

pantothenic acid, 56
papules, 11, 34
peels, 68–70, 81, 88
penicillin, 63
peroxide see benzoyl peroxide
perspiration, 44
pH balance, skin, 72
phones, cleaning, 27
pigmentation, 35, 73, 78, 83
pigments, skin care products, 31
polycystic ovary disease, 19
pore strips, 30
pores, clogging, 30–1
powder, 39

Prednisone, 63
pregnancy, 12, 21, 67
prescription drugs, 60–7
progesterone, 18
Progionibacterium acnes
  (P. acnes), 13, 50, 62
pseudo scars, 78
puberty, 12
punch excision, scar removal, 83
pustules, 11, 34
pyridoxine, 56

raised scars, 79
resourcinol, 51
Retin-A®, 60
retinoids, 64, 67, 72, 89
rhinophyma, 88
rosacea, 85–91

salicylic acid, 21, 45, 51, 70
scars, 34, 35, 38, 77–83
sebaceous glands, 9, 12–13, 44
sebum, 9, 12
skin: cleansing, 24, 26
  skin care products, 28–31
soap, 24
Spironolactone, 63
squeezing spots, 34–5, 40
staphylococci, 34
steam cleansing, 40, 41
steroids, 13, 52, 89
streptococci, 34
stress, 16
subcision, scar removal, 83
sugars, 31
sulfa, 63

sulfacetamide, 65
sulfur, 51, 65
sulfur/resourcinol, 51
sun exposure, 43, 67, 78
sunscreens, 33, 43, 67
surgery, scar removal, 83
sweat, 44
sweat bumps, 85

T-zone, 26
tazarotene, 65
tea tree oil, 55
telephones, cleaning, 27
testosterone, 13
tetracyclines, 62, 63
thromycin, 65
tretinoin, 65, 89
trichloracetic acid, 70, 81
ultraviolet light, 43

vasodilator drugs, 89
vitamins, 31
vitamin A derivatives, 20, 21,
  43, 57, 60, 64, 67, 72
vitamin B3, 57
vitamin B5, 56
vitamin B6, 56

water, drinking, 23
waxes, 31
whiteheads, 10, 34
  extracting, 40, 41
wrinkles, 72

zinc, 56

acknowledgments

Special thanks to my gorgeous girl Eden Claire for giving me a reason to write. My great appreciation goes to Alison Cathie and Jane O'Shea for having a vision, and to Lisa Pendreigh and Katie Ginn for making it work.

I also wish to thank the many doctors, surgeons and experts who kindly gave their time and shared their knowledge with me to help with my research. Albert Lefkovits, Nicholas Lowe, Seth Matarasso, Laurie Polis, David J. Goldberg, Roy Geronemus, Harold Brody, Kenneth Beer, Diane Berson.

picture credits

For more information on complexion perfection visit Wendy Lewis's website at www.wlbeauty.com or email your skin care queries to wlbeauty@aol.com.